RECTAL SURGERY RECOVERY NUTRITION

Complete Guide Unlocking The Secrets Of
Nutrition To Rapid Healing After Surgery
Success, Nourishing Meal Plans, Recipes, Tips
For Optimal Health Wellness

DR. ALLAN FREDA

Contents

INTRODUCTION

Welcome to this complete guide on what to eat after having rectal surgery. After having rectal surgery, this recipe is meant to help you heal by giving you useful information and useful recommendations. We know that the healing process can be hard on you, both physically and emotionally. However good nutrition is a key part of speeding up the healing process, preventing complications, and improving your general health. This guide is designed to help people who are recovering from rectal surgery. It includes expert tips, healing recipes, meal plans, and long-term health strategies.

This cookbook is about:

The experts who put together this cookbook, which included nutritionists, dietitians, and surgeons, used scientific proof to advise on how to eat after surgery.

Its goal is to give you the information and tools you need to make smart food choices that will help you recover and improve your health.

For people who have just been diagnosed or who are caring for a loved one and want to help them through their healing, this guide will help you understand the complicated world of nutrition after surgery.

Nutrition is very important for getting better after having stomach surgery. No matter what kind of surgery it is, it puts the body under a lot of stress, which causes metabolic and immune reactions that help the body heal and repair tissues.

To support these processes and ensure the best possible recovery outcomes, it is important to get enough nutrition. For people who are going to have rectal surgery, good nutrition is even more important because of the unique challenges and needs of the operation.

Keeping up a healthy caloric intake:

After rectal surgery, your body may need more energy as it works to heal tissues and get back to normal physiological processes. To meet these higher energy needs and avoid malnutrition, it is important to keep up a healthy caloric diet.

It may be hard to eat enough calories, though, because of things like pain, sickness, and changes in desire. Focusing on foods that are high in nutrients and eating smaller meals or snacks more often can help make sure that your body gets the energy and nutrients it needs to heal.

Getting the Most Protein:

Protein is an important nutrient for healing after surgery because it helps fix tissues, heal wounds, and keep the immune system working well.

Protein needs may be higher after rectal surgery to help the body make new tissues and speed up the mending process.

To meet these higher needs, you must eat a lot of high-quality protein sources, like lean meats, chicken, fish, eggs, dairy products, legumes, and nuts. Protein-rich drinks like smoothies and protein shakes can be a handy way to get more protein if you have trouble eating solid foods.

Equilibrium of Macronutrients:

Along with protein, it is important to make sure that your food after surgery has the right amount of carbs and fats. For your body, carbohydrates are the main source of energy, and fats help make hormones, absorb nutrients, and keep cell membranes strong. Complex carbs, like those found in whole grains, fruits, and veggies, can help keep blood sugar levels steady and give you energy all day. In the same way, eating healthy fats like those found in avocados, olive oil, nuts, and seeds can help keep your body's nutrition in balance and support many biological processes.

Getting enough water and fluids:

Staying hydrated is important for healing after surgery because it helps keep the body's fluid balance, control temperature, and support cell function. Being dehydrated can slow down the mending process and raise the risk of problems like urinary tract infections and constipation.

During the day, try to drink a lot of water, herbal teas, broths, and drinks that are high in electrolytes. But be careful not to drink too much coffee or sugary drinks, as they can make you pee more, which could make you even more dehydrated.

Fibre and Having Regular Bowels:

After rectal surgery, it's important to keep up with normal bowel movements to avoid problems like constipation and fecal impaction. Getting enough fiber is a key part of keeping your bowels normal and avoiding constipation after surgery.

But it's important to slowly eat more fiber and pick foods that are easy on the digestive system, like whole grains, fruits, veggies, and legumes. Make sure to drink a lot of water and eat foods that are high in fiber to help soften your stools and make them easier to pass through your bowels.

Supplements for nutrition:

It can be hard to get all the nutrients you need from food alone, especially at the beginning of your healing when you may not be hungry or able to handle solid foods well. In these cases, vitamin supplements may be suggested to make up the difference and make sure the body gets enough of the nutrients it needs.

Depending on your nutritional needs and healing goals, your doctor may tell you to take certain supplements. Protein powders, vitamin and mineral supplements, probiotics, and special enteral nutrition mixes are some of the supplements that may be used.

Making a Plate Full of Nutrients:

When making meals for recovery after abdominal surgery, try to make a plate with a lot of different foods from different food groups. A well-balanced meal should have a lean protein source, like fish or chicken breast that has been baked, and a lot of different coloured fruits and veggies.

Whole grains, like quinoa or brown rice, can give you complex carbs and fiber. Healthy fats, like those found in avocado or olive oil, can help you feel full and absorb nutrients better.

Some ideas for meals:

• For breakfast, I had a Greek yogurt parfait with cereal and fresh berries.

For lunch, I had grilled salmon salad with mixed veggies, avocado, and balsamic vinaigrette.

As for dinner, I had roasted chicken breast with rice pilaf and steamed broccoli.

• Snacks: apple slices with almond butter, hummus on carrot sticks, or a protein shake made with spinach, banana, and protein powder.

Changing the consistency and texture:

Depending on your food habits and level of tolerance after surgery, you may need to change the texture and consistency of your meals to make them easier to swallow and digest.

During the early stages of recovery, soft, pureed, or liquid-based foods may be better accepted.

As tolerance grows, firmer textures can be added. Try making meals in different ways, like slow cooking, blending, or steaming, to make meals that are healthy and easy to digest.

Adding Ingredients That Heal:

Some foods and products are known to help the body heal, so adding them to your diet after surgery can be helpful.

Berries, leafy greens, and colorful veggies are all examples of foods that are high in antioxidants and can help reduce inflammation and speed up tissue repair. Fish with a lot of omega-3 fatty acids, flaxseeds, and walnuts may help wounds heal by reducing inflammation. Adding herbs and spices like garlic, turmeric, and ginger can also make food taste better and may be good for you.

Tips from experts for long-term health

Patience and Gradual Progress:

Rectal surgery recovery is a slow process that needs patience and persistence. Instead of rushing back to your normal diet, it's important to pay attention to your body's signals and slowly add foods back in as allowed. Start with small amounts of food and slowly increase the size of your meals and the types of food you eat as your tolerance grows.

Be kind to yourself and believe that your body will heal and get stronger with time and steady effort.

Speaking with medical experts:

Keep the lines of communication open with your healthcare team, which includes your surgeon, dietitian, and other allied health workers as you recover.

They can give you personalised advice and help based on your needs and how well you are recovering. Please don't be afraid to ask for help if you have any worrying signs or problems with your diet. Your healthcare providers are there to help you get better and make sure the best results are achieved.

Eating mindfully and feeling good about yourself:

It can help your physical and mental health during the recovery process to incorporate mindfulness practices into the way you eat. Pay attention to your body's signals for when you're hungry or full, and savor each bite by focusing on how it feels in your mouth.

Use relaxation methods like deep breathing, meditation, or gentle stretching to lower your stress and feel more at ease. Remember that healing is more than just getting better physically. It also entails looking after your emotional and mental well-being.

Disclaimer

The information in this book is for informational purposes only and should not replace professional medical advice, diagnosis, or treatment. Always consult your physician or a qualified health provider regarding any medical concerns. Do not disregard professional medical advice or delay seeking it based on information in this book.

The author does not endorse or have affiliations with any mentioned entities. References are for informational purposes only.

Consult your healthcare provider before making dietary or lifestyle changes, especially during recovery from surgery, as individual needs vary.

Results may vary, and the information provided is not guaranteed to produce specific outcomes.

By reading this book, you acknowledge and agree to consult your healthcare provider before implementing any information herein.

For further guidance, consult your healthcare provider or reputable medical websites for reliable information on surgery recovery diets.

CHAPTER 1
GETTING READY FOR SURGERY

Rectal surgery, which is also sometimes called colorectal surgery, includes several procedures that are used to address problems with the rectum and colon. You might need these treatments to fix problems like colorectal cancer, inflammatory bowel disease (IBD), diverticulitis, rectal prolapse, or other issues with the structure of your body. According to the underlying condition, the goal of rectal surgery can be different, but it usually involves getting rid of diseased tissue, fixing or rebuilding damaged areas, or relieving symptoms like pain, bleeding, or blockage.

Before getting into the specifics of recovery diet, it's important to know what rectal surgery is and how it affects the body.

Rectal surgery is often a major treatment that needs to be done in the hospital and requires a long time to recover from. It could be open surgery, minimally invasive methods like laparoscopy, or surgery with robotic help.

Each has its own set of issues to think about and risks that could happen. Patients who have rectal surgery may have temporary or lasting changes in how their bowels work, such as changes in their bowel habits, the consistency of their stools, and how often they go to the toilet. Having surgery can also put stress on the body, which can cause it to use more energy, need more nutrients, and have higher metabolic demands while it heals.

Getting your kitchen ready:

Getting ready for healing from rectal surgery starts a long time before the surgery itself. Make sure your kitchen has everything you need to meet your food needs while you're healing. This is an important part of getting ready.

A well-stocked kitchen can make it easier to follow dietary guidelines, make healthy meals, and stay hydrated, all of which are important for healing and recovering as quickly as possible. Here are some important things you can do to get your kitchen ready for food after surgery:

First, get rid of any processed or unhealthy foods that are in your cupboard, fridge, and freezer. Instead, eat foods that are high in nutrients, like fruits, veggies, whole grains, lean proteins, and healthy fats. Having healthy foods on hand will make it easier to make well-balanced meals that help with healing and general health.

Get kitchen tools and equipment that make it easier to make meals, like a food processor or blender for making smoothies or pureed foods, a slow cooker for making healthy soups and stews, and storage containers for dividing up meals and snacks.

These tools can speed up the cooking process and make it easier to handle, especially if you are still recovering and don't have much energy or movement.

Get extra of the things you need in the pantry that last a long time and are easy to use in meals and snacks. Some examples are whole grain pasta or rice, low-sodium soup or stock, nut butter, dried fruits and nuts, and herbs and spices that add flavor to food without adding salt or sugar.

Knowing you have these basic items on hand will give you a range of choices when planning and making meals, even if you can't go shopping often or get fresh food.

You might want to prepare and freeze meals ahead of time so that you have ready-to-eat choices when you're still recovering and finding it hard to cook. Pick recipes that are high in nutrients, easy to stomach, and can be easily divided into servings for each person. When it comes to freezer-friendly meals that can be enjoyed quickly with little work, soups, casseroles, and smoothie packs are great choices.

Planning your meals is an important part of nutrition after surgery because it helps you eat a healthy diet that meets your body's higher nutrient needs while it heals. Meal planning can also help you feel less stressed, save you time when you go food shopping, and help you follow the dietary advice your healthcare team gives you. Here are some tips for planning meals well while you're recovering from rectal surgery:

Talk to a registered dietitian or nutritionist to make a personalized meal plan that takes into account your individual nutritional needs, food preferences, and any dietary restrictions or changes that your surgery or underlying medical condition requires. You can get personalised advice and support from a trained nutritionist to help you make the most of your diet for healing and recovery.

Focus on eating a wide range of healthy foods at meals and snacks, such as whole grains, fruits, veggies, lean proteins, and healthy fats. To help heal wounds and fix tissues, try to eat protein-rich foods with every meal. These could be chicken, fish, tofu, beans, eggs, or dairy products.

Whole grains, fruits, veggies, legumes, and other high-fiber carbs are good for your digestive health and regularity. Refined grains and added sugars, on the other hand, can cause inflammation and stomach pain.

Controlling your portions will help you stay healthy and not overeat while you're recovering. Watch out for signs that you're hungry or full, and try to eat healthy meals and snacks at regular times throughout the day to keep your energy up and help your body heal. To help control serving sizes, use smaller plates and utensils, and don't eat straight from containers or packages, which can make you eat without thinking and take in too many calories.

Drink a lot of water, herbal tea, broth-based soups, and fruit drinks that have been diluted throughout the day to stay hydrated. Staying hydrated is important for wound healing, keeping your intestines moving, and your general health and well-being. At least eight cups of fluid should be drunk every day. If you're busy or losing more fluids than usual because of things like fever, sweating, or diarrhea, drink even more.

Try out different ways to cook and combine flavors to keep meals interesting and fun, even if you are following dietary guidelines or limits. You can bring out the natural flavors and textures of foods by grilling, roasting, steaming, sautéing, or baking them. You can also add extra flavor without adding salt or sugar by seasoning meals with herbs, spices, citrus juices, and vinegar. You can make changes and substitutions to recipes in creative ways to meet your nutritional needs and help your body heal if you have any food allergies or preferences.

To help your body heal after rectal surgery, eat and snack on foods and items that are good for you. Vitamin C-rich fruits and vegetables, zinc-rich foods like lean meats and seafood, omega-3 fatty acids found in fatty fish, flaxseeds, and walnuts, and phytonutrient-rich herbs and spices like turmeric, ginger, garlic, and cinnamon are just a few examples of foods that can help your body heal wounds, reduce inflammation, and keep your immune system strong.

Try therapeutic foods and supplements that may help ease common problems or symptoms that come up after surgery. For example, probiotics can help restore the balance of gut flora and stop diarrhea or constipation, prebiotic fibers can help your digestive health and immune system work better, and collagen peptides or amino acid supplements can help your body heal and repair damaged tissues. Before starting any new supplements, talk to your doctor, especially if you are already on medications or have a health problem that could affect how the supplements work for you.

Mindful eating can improve your general eating experience, help your digestion, make you feel full, and make you more aware of when you're hungry or full. Slow down and chew your food well to help your body digest it and avoid pain or bloating.

Also, turn off screens during meals and focus on the sensory aspects of eating, like the smell, taste, and feel of food. Pay attention to your body's cues about hunger and fullness, and stop eating when you're pleased, not too full.

During the recovery time, ask family, friends, or carers to help you with things like making meals, grocery shopping, and housework. As you heal from rectal surgery, don't be afraid to give tasks to other people or ask for help when you need it. Keeping up with daily tasks and responsibilities may be hard. Self-care and rest should be your top priorities, and you should focus on feeding and drinking healthy foods and drinks to help your body heal and speed up your recovery.

By using these tips and tricks, you can make the most of your post-surgery food to help you heal, lower your risk of complications, and improve your health and well-being in general while you're recovering. Remember to talk to your healthcare team about your specific needs and medical background to get personalized advice and suggestions. Also, don't be afraid to ask for help if you have questions or concerns about your diet or recovery progress. By taking care of yourself and eating right, you can make your healing from rectal surgery go more smoothly and improve your health in the long run.

CHAPTER 2
FOODS THAT ARE HIGH IN NUTRIENTS

When it comes to eating for recovering from rectal surgery, knowing the importance of nutrient-rich ingredients is very important. These ingredients must help the body heal by repairing tissues, increasing the immune system, and replacing nutrients that were lost during surgery. Recovery and general health need to eat a range of whole foods that are high in vitamins, minerals, antioxidants, and other helpful compounds.

How to Add Whole Foods:

Fruits, veggies, whole grains, lean proteins, nuts, seeds, and legumes are just a few of the naturally nutrient-dense foods that are considered whole. These foods have not been processed or have been processed very little. They have kept their original nutritional value and offer many health benefits.

By eating whole foods after surgery, you can get a wide range of vitamins, minerals, fiber, and phytonutrients that are important for helping your body heal. Antioxidants are found in large amounts in fruits and vegetables.

They help lower inflammation, fight oxidative stress, and speed up the healing of tissues. Whole grains like oats, quinoa, and brown rice are great sources of complex carbohydrates, which give you the energy that lasts and helps your body digest food. Lean proteins, like those found in chicken, fish, tofu, and lentils, are important for building muscle and keeping your immune system healthy. People who have recently had surgery can get the most nutrients out of their diet and heal faster by focusing on whole foods.

Important Nutrients for Healing:

Some foods are very important for getting better after having rectal surgery. Some of these are copper, omega-3 fatty acids, fiber, protein, vitamin

C, vitamin A, and vitamin C. Protein is necessary for wound healing and muscle repair, so it's also important for recovery after surgery. To meet your higher protein needs during this time, you should eat lean protein sources like chicken, turkey, fish, eggs, tofu, and beans at every meal.

Vitamin C is a strong vitamin that helps the immune system work and makes collagen, which helps wounds heal and tissues grow back.

Citrus fruits, strawberries, bell peppers, broccoli, and kiwi are all foods that are high in vitamin C.

Vitamin A helps the skin and immune system work well, which lowers the risk of getting infections and speeds up the healing of wounds. Carrots, sweet potatoes, spinach, kale, and liver are all good sources of vitamin A. Zinc is needed for the defence system, making proteins, and healing wounds. Whole grains, meat, shellfish, seeds, and nuts are all good sources of zinc. Omega-3 fatty acids are found in fatty fish, flaxseeds, chia seeds, and peanuts. They help keep your heart healthy and reduce inflammation. Lastly, fiber is found in lots of fruits, vegetables, whole grains, and legumes. It helps digestion, keeps bowels regular, and avoids constipation. Making sure you get enough of these important nutrients is important for helping your body heal and get better after surgery.

Things you should not eat:

Focusing on nutrient-dense foods is important for healing after surgery, but it's also important to be aware of foods that may slow down the healing process or make conditions worse.

During the recovery time, you should limit or avoid certain foods and drinks to keep you from getting too sick or hurt and to help your body heal as quickly as possible. High-fat and fried foods may make stomach problems worse and raise the risk of having gut problems like diarrhea or constipation. Foods that are spicy or high in added sugars or artificial sweeteners can irritate the digestive system and make problems like gas, bloating, or stomach pain worse. Limit your intake of caffeinated, alcoholic, and fizzy drinks as well, since they can make you dehydrated, mess up your medications, and make your stomach work less well.

Processed foods that are high in salt, artificial additives, and preservatives should be avoided because they are not very healthy and may slow down the body's healing processes. People who are recovering from rectal surgery should also talk to their doctor or a registered dietitian about what they should eat based on their needs, medical background, and any other conditions they may have. People who have had rectal surgery can speed up their recovery and improve their health in the long run by avoiding certain foods and focusing on foods that are high in nutrients.

CHAPTER 3
SOUPS AND BREADS THAT HEAL

In terms of nutrition for recovering from rectal surgery, eating healing soups and broths is very important for speeding up the healing process and improving general health. These liquid foods are good for you in many ways, like making processing easier, keeping you hydrated, and giving you the nutrients, your body needs to repair tissues and keep your immune system strong. This detailed guide goes into great detail about the importance of healing soups and broths, looking at different kinds and how they can help you.

Healthy Bone Broths

Because it is full of nutrients and helps the body heal, bone broth is an important part of the diet after surgery. Bone broth is made by boiling animal bones and connective tissues in water for a long time. It is full of minerals like calcium and magnesium, amino acids, collagen, and gelatin, all of which are important for healing tissues, keeping bones strong, and keeping your gut healthy. Collagen, which is found in large amounts in bone broth, helps cuts heal and tissues grow back.

This makes it an important part of diets for people who have recently had surgery. Also, the amino acids in bone broth, like glycine and proline, help reduce inflammation, which speeds up the healing process considerably. Including healthy bone broths in your diet after having abdominal surgery can help with healing and recovery by giving your body back the nutrients it needs for long-term health.

Soups made with vegetables

Adding vegetable-based soups to your diet after surgery can help your health in many ways, from giving you more nutrients to boosting your immune system. These soups are made from many different nutrient-dense veggies.

They are full of vitamins, minerals, antioxidants, and fiber, all of which are important for health and healing. Cruciferous veggies, like broccoli, cauliflower, and Brussels sprouts, are full of sulfur-containing compounds that help the body get rid of toxins and reduce inflammation.

This makes them especially good for people who have recently had surgery and are still recovering. Also, veggies like kale, spinach, and carrots are full of vitamins A, C, and K, which are very important for healing wounds, making collagen, and keeping your immune system strong. By adding a variety of veggies to soups, people who are having rectal surgery can make sure they get all the nutrients they need and help their bodies heal properly.

Stews Full of Protein

Protein is an important nutrient for healing after surgery because it helps fix tissues, keep muscles strong, and keep the immune system working well. Stews that are high in protein are an easy and tasty way to get the extra protein you need while you are healing from rectal surgery.

 By adding lean meats, poultry, fish, or plant-based protein sources like beans and lentils to hearty stews, you can make sure you get enough of the important amino acids your body needs to heal wounds and grow new tissues.

Adding herbs, spices, and veggies to stews not only makes them taste better, but they also add a lot of micronutrients and phytochemicals that are good for your health and well-being. By making protein-rich stews a priority in their post-surgery meal plans, people can speed up their recovery, keep their muscle mass, and improve their health in the long run.

To sum up, healing soups and broths, such as bone broths, veggie soups, and stews full of protein, are very important for speeding up the healing process after rectal surgery.

These liquid foods are high in nutrients and easy to digest. They give you essential nutrients, help your body heal, and improve your general health.

By eating a range of healing soups and broths, people can improve their nutrition after surgery, speed up the healing process, and set themselves up for long-term health and vitality.

CHAPTER 4
DISHES THAT ARE SOFT AND EASY TO DIGEST

When it comes to eating for recovering from rectal surgery, soft, easy-to-digest foods are very important. The goal of this diet plan is to give patients healthy meals that are easy on the digestive system but full of nutrients that are important for healing and general health. After surgery, there is a very important time when the body needs the best diet to help heal tissues, reduce inflammation, and boost immune function. Because of this, adding soft, easily edible foods to the diet can help the healing process a lot.

Many types of meals are soft and easy to digest, such as mild grain dishes, creamy polenta and porridge, and mashed vegetable creations. There are different health benefits in each of these groups, and they can all be changed to fit different tastes and food needs.

By learning about the meanings behind these foods and how they help with recovery after surgery, patients can make choices that will help them get better.

Comfort food made with whole grains is a great way to get carbs, which are important for giving the body energy while it heals. Rice, quinoa, and couscous are all examples of gentle grains because they can all be cooked until they are soft and easy to stomach. These foods don't have a lot of fiber, so they're easy on the digestive system and good for people who are sensitive or in pain after surgery. Herbs, spices, and mild sauces can also be added to mild-grain meals to make them taste better and add more nutrition.

Creamy polenta and porridge are warming and healthy foods that have a soft texture and help the digestive system feel better. Polenta is made from cornmeal and can be cooked until it's creamy.

It can then be used as a base for many different toppings, like sautéed veggies, grilled protein, or savory sauces. In the same way, you can cook porridge with milk or water to make a creamy and filling meal. Porridge is usually made from oats or other grains. These dishes are great for people who are healing from rectal surgery because they are high in carbs, fiber, and important nutrients.

Making mashed vegetable dishes is a healthy and easy-to-digest alternative to eating whole veggies, which can be hard for some people to handle after surgery. You can boil or steam vegetables like potatoes, carrots, squash, and peas until they are soft, then mash or puree them to make smooth, tasty meals. Vegetable dishes made with mashed potatoes are full of vitamins, minerals, and antioxidants that help the immune system work well and help tissues heal.

You can also add herbs, spices, and healthy fats like avocado or olive oil to these meals to make them taste better and make them healthier.

Finally, foods that are soft and easy to digest are very important for people who have had rectal surgery because they help them recover by giving them healthy meals that are easy on the digestive system but full of important nutrients.

Gentle grain dishes, creamy polenta and porridge, and mashed vegetable creations give people a lot of choices to meet their tastes and dietary needs. Patients can help their healing process and promote long-term health by adding these foods to their post-surgery diet.

CHAPTER 5
MEALS PACKED WITH PROTEIN

When it comes to diet for recovering from rectal surgery, protein is very important. Getting enough protein is important for healing wounds, repairing tissues, and getting better generally. This part will talk about how important it is to eat foods that are high in protein and look at different plant-based and lean protein sources. We will also talk about how important it is to balance macronutrients for the best healing.

Sources of Lean Protein

Lean protein sources are very important for people who have had rectal surgery because they give the body the building blocks it needs to mend and grow new tissue without adding too much-saturated fat. Skinless chicken and turkey breast, lean cuts of beef and pork, fish, eggs, and low-fat dairy products like Greek yogurt and cottage cheese are all good sources of lean protein. These high-protein foods not only help the body heal, but they also help keep muscle mass, which can be lost during times when you can't move around or do as much physical exercise after surgery. Including lean protein in snacks and meals throughout the day can help make sure you get enough amino acids, which are the building blocks of protein, to heal properly.

There are many protein-rich foods to choose from for people who are vegetarian or vegan or just want to eat more plant-based foods. Beans, lentils, and chickpeas are all legumes that are great plant-based sources of protein that can be added to salads, soups, and stews. You can also use tofu, tempeh, and soybeans as plant-based sources of protein in a variety of ways, such as in stir-fries, sandwiches, or traditional recipes instead of meat. Nuts and seeds, like almonds, walnuts, chia seeds, and hemp seeds, also have protein and healthy fats, which makes them great for snacks or adding to yogurt and salads. By eating a wide range of plant-based foods and different types of protein, people can meet their protein needs and also enjoy the benefits of a healthy diet that is high in fiber, vitamins, and minerals.

For the best healing after abdominal surgery, it is important to balance macronutrients, which include carbs and fats, as well as getting enough protein. As the body's main source of energy, carbohydrates are important for keeping cells running and allowing people to be active.

Choose complex carbs like whole grains, fruits, veggies, and legumes. They give you long-lasting energy and important nutrients like minerals, vitamins, and fiber. Eating healthy fats like those found in eggs, olive oil, nuts, and seeds can help lower inflammation and keep cells working well.

Aim for a mix of carbs, protein, and fats in each meal and snack to help you feel full, keep your blood sugar levels stable, and help your body heal and recover overall.

people who have had rectal surgery need to eat a lot of protein-rich foods because they give their bodies the nutrients, they need to repair tissue, heal wounds, and get better overall.

To meet your daily protein needs, you should eat lean protein sources like chicken, fish, eggs, dairy products, and nuts, as well as plant-based protein sources like beans, tofu, and seeds. Including complex carbohydrates, healthy fats, and protein in a balanced macronutrient diet can help with healing and promote long-term health.

People can improve their nutrition after surgery and general health and well-being by focusing on nutrient-rich foods and eating a variety of foods.

CHAPTER 6
RECIPES THAT ARE GOOD FOR YOU

When you're recovering from rectal surgery, you need to pay close attention to what you eat because it can have a big effect on how quickly you heal. This detailed guide aims to teach you important things about a fiber-friendly diet after having abdominal surgery, such as how to slowly add fiber back into your diet, high-fiber fruit and vegetable dishes, fiber supplements, and other choices.

Reintroducing fiber slowly:

It's important to slowly add fiber back into your diet after stomach surgery. Fibre is important for digestive health and normal bowel movements, but if you eat too much of it too soon, it can make it harder for your digestive system to heal. Start with low-fiber foods that are easy to digest, like cooked veggies, fruits that have been peeled, and refined grains. As your body gets used to these foods, slowly add more fiber by eating more whole grains, legumes, and fibrous fruits and veggies. This slow method lets your digestive system get used to the changes and avoids any pain or problems that might happen.

Fruit and vegetable dishes that are high in fiber: Adding fruits and veggies high in fiber to your diet after surgery can help you heal and stay regular while giving you important nutrients. If you want to be easy on your stomach, choose cooking soft fruits, like applesauce, mashed bananas, and stewed prunes. Carrots, squash, potatoes, and other vegetables can be steamed or roasted until soft, which makes them easier to swallow. You can also sauté or mix leafy greens like spinach and kale into soups to add more fiber and nutrients.

Try out different cooking methods and recipes to make tasty, high-fiber meals that will help you on your way to recovery.

It might be hard to get all the fibre you need from food alone, especially when you are first starting to feel better. Fibre products can be helpful after surgery because they make it easy to get more fiber without making you feel bulky or uncomfortable. Options like acacia fiber, psyllium husk, and methylcellulose are often used and come in different forms, such as powders, pills, and chewable tablets. Before taking any fiber supplements, you should talk to your doctor to make sure they are right for you and won't get in the way of your recovery. You can also get soluble fiber from foods like oats, chia seeds, and flaxseeds instead of pills. These foods can be added to smoothies, oatmeal, or baked goods to give them an extra fiber boost.

To sum up, a diet high in fiber is important for getting better after stomach surgery. You can help your body heal and improve your digestive health in the long run by slowly adding fiber back into your diet, eating more high-fiber fruits and vegetables, and thinking about fiber supplements and other options. Always pay attention to what your body is telling you and work together with your healthcare team to make sure your diet fits your needs and tastes. You can get your body healthy again and live a fulfilling life after surgery if you are patient and mindful, and make healthy choices.

CHAPTER 7
ELECTROLYTES AND WATER

Hydration and electrolytes are very important for getting better after rectal surgery. Keeping your body's processes going, helping it heal, and avoiding problems all depend on having the right amount of water and electrolytes. In this part, we'll talk about why staying hydrated is important, how to replace electrolytes, and some ideas for drinks that will help you stay hydrated and recover.

Getting enough water is very important for healing after rectal surgery. Making sure you drink enough water helps your body do many important things that are needed for healing, like getting nutrients to cells, getting rid of trash, keeping your body temperature stable, and many other things. Dehydration can slow down recovery by lowering blood flow, making it harder for wounds to heal, and raising the risk of problems like urinary tract infections and nausea.

So, keeping your body at the right level of hydration is essential for recovery and general health.

During the recovery time, it's just as important to replace electrolytes. Electrolytes are chemicals like sodium, potassium, calcium, and magnesium that help keep the body's fluid balance, keep nerves and muscles working, and keep blood pressure in check. Stress from surgery, fluid loss through drainage tubes, and changes in bowel habits are all things that can throw off the balance of electrolytes. Adding minerals back into the body helps restore balance, keep you from becoming dehydrated, and keep your body working at its best while you're recovering.

To make sure you stay hydrated and replace your electrolytes, it's important to include a variety of refreshing drinks in your diet after surgery. Here are some ideas for drinks that will keep you hydrated and help you recover:

1. To stay hydrated, plain water is the most basic and important drink. To stay hydrated, encourage sipping often throughout the day.

2. Electrolyte-enhanced drinks: Electrolyte drinks or oral rehydration solutions that you can buy can help you get back the fluids you lost during surgery and stay hydrated. But watch out for extra sugars and choose sugar-free or low-sugar options when you can.

3. Coconut water: Coconut water naturally has a lot of electrolytes, especially potassium, which makes it a great way to stay hydrated and replace lost electrolytes. It's also cooling and easy on the stomach, so it's good for people who are recovering from surgery.

4. Herbal teas: Chamomile, ginger, peppermint, and other non-caffeinated herbal teas can help you stay hydrated and are also good for you.

These drinks can help calm the stomach, stop nausea, and make you feel more relaxed, all of which can help you while you're healing.

5. Broth: Clear broth made from bones, veggies, or lean meats can be a healthy and hydrating choice after surgery. Broth not only keeps you hydrated, but it also gives you important nutrients like protein, vitamins, and minerals that help your body heal and get better.

6. Fruit juices: Apple or grape juice, which has been diluted, can serve as a source of water natural sugars, and vitamins. But it's important to pick juices that are 100% pure and don't have any extra sugars. Also, because they have a lot of sugar, you should only drink them in moderation.

Adding a range of hydrating drinks to your diet after surgery can help you stay properly hydrated, replace lost electrolytes, and speed up the healing process. Encourage people to sip often throughout the day, and make sure that everyone can find a drink that suits their tastes and limits.

You should also talk to a doctor or trained dietitian to get personalised advice based on your specific dietary needs and the needs of the surgery.

People who are having rectal surgery can speed up their healing and improve their long-term health by putting hydration and electrolyte balance first.

CHAPTER 8
SNACKS AND DESSERTS THAT HEAL

Healing snacks and desserts are very important for nutrition during and after rectal surgery because they provide important nutrients to help the body heal and also make the person feel good during the recovery time. This part talks about how important it is to include nutrient-dense treats, low-sugar desserts, and filling snack ideas in your diet after surgery to help you heal better and stay healthy in the long run.

Nutrient-Dense Treats: Nutrient-dense treats are an important part of nutrition for people recovering from rectal surgery because they give the body the vitamins, minerals, and enzymes it needs to heal tissues and keep the immune system working well. Choose treats that are high in nutrients like zinc, omega-3 fatty acids, vitamins A, C, and E.

This will help you heal faster and lower your risk of problems. As examples of treats that are high in nutrients, fresh fruits like berries are high in vitamins, nuts, and seeds are high in healthy fats and protein, and dark chocolate has flavonoids that are known to reduce inflammation.

Not only do these treats satisfy your needs, but they also help your health and well-being while you're recovering.

Low-Sugar Desserts: It's especially important to choose low-sugar desserts while recovering from rectal surgery since too much sugar can make inflammation worse and slow down the healing process. People who are recovering from rectal surgery don't have to eat traditional desserts that are high in sugar.

Instead, they can choose healthier desserts that please their sweet tooth without making their blood sugar levels rise. Some sweet desserts without adding sugar are sugar-free jelly, homemade fruit sorbets sweetened with natural sweeteners like stevia or monk fruit, and yogurt parfait with fresh fruits and a drizzle of honey. These desserts are low in sugar, which helps keep blood sugar levels steady and improves recovery after surgery.

Satisfying Snack Ideas: Adding satisfying snack ideas to your diet after surgery is important for keeping your energy up and stopping you from feeling too hungry in between meals.

Snacks should have a good mix of protein, healthy fats, and complex carbs to help keep blood sugar levels steady and make you feel full. Whole grain crackers with hummus or avocado, Greek yogurt with nuts and seeds, vegetable sticks with guacamole or nut butter, and homemade trail mix with dried fruits and raw nuts are all tasty snacks that can help you feel better after having rectal surgery. Not only do these snacks give people important nutrients, but they also help them stay happy and fed while they're healing.

Also, picking snacks that are easy to digest can help with stomach problems and speed up the healing process after surgery.

It is important to include healing snacks and desserts in your diet after surgery to help you recover quickly and stay healthy in the long run. People can help their bodies heal, keep their blood sugar levels stable, and avoid nutritional deficits while they are recovering by focusing on treats that are high in nutrients, desserts that are low in sugar, and satisfying snack ideas. Talking to a doctor or registered dietitian can also help you make a nutrition plan for after surgery that fits your needs and tastes. This will help you recover faster and be healthier overall.

CHAPTER 9
USING HERBS AND SPICES FOR HEALTH

Including healing herbs and spices in your diet while you are recovering from surgery can speed up the healing process and improve your general health. These natural ingredients are good for you in many ways, from reducing inflammation to improving digestion and making food taste better. To speed up recovery and promote long-term health, it's important to know what these parts mean and how to use them correctly.

Ingredients that reduce inflammation:

When the body is hurt or traumatized, including during surgery, it naturally reacts with inflammation. However, too much inflammation can slow down the mending process and cause problems.

Adding anti-inflammatory foods to your diet can help reduce inflammation and speed up the body's mending processes.

Curcumin, the main ingredient in turmeric, is known for its powerful ability to reduce inflammation. It can be added to many foods or taken on its own as a supplement to help the body heal and prevent inflammation. In the same way, ginger has gingerol in it, a bioactive substance that has anti-inflammatory and antioxidant properties that make it a good food to eat after surgery.

You can find omega-3 fatty acids in flaxseeds and fatty foods like salmon. These acids help lower inflammation and control how the body reacts to it. Adding these things to your diet can help reduce swelling and speed up the healing process.

There are a lot of vitamins and phytonutrients that fight inflammation in dark leafy greens like spinach and kale.

You can eat these veggies raw in salads or cooked as part of healthy meals to help reduce inflammation.

Anesthesia and surgery can sometimes mess up the digestive system, which can cause problems like nausea or bloating. Digestive aid plants can help ease these symptoms and keep your digestive system healthy while you're healing.

Peppermint is a well-known plant that can help with stomach problems like indigestion, gas, and nausea. Having peppermint tea or putting fresh mint leaves on food can help you feel better and keep your digestive system working well.

There are chemicals in fennel seeds that help relax the digestive system and lower gas and bloating. Adding fennel seeds to food or drinking fennel tea can help your body digest food and calm your stomach.

Chamomile is another herb that is known to help the digestive system.

Its anti-inflammatory and calming qualities can ease digestive pain. Chamomile tea can help you relax and digest food better when you drink it after a meal.

Improving the taste of food after surgery is important for keeping your appetite and making sure you get enough nutrition. Spice mixes not only make food taste better, but they are also good for you in many ways, so they are a great addition to a recovery diet.

Cinnamon is a useful spice that can be used to make food warmer and sweeter. It can also help control blood sugar and reduce swelling. Adding cinnamon to smoothies or topping muesli with it can make them taste better and be better for you.

Capsaicin, which is found in cayenne pepper, is a chemical that is known to relieve pain and speed up the metabolism.

Adding a pinch of cayenne to savory foods can give them a tasty kick while also helping with healing and health in general.

People love garlic for its unique flavor and many health benefits, such as its ability to reduce inflammation and improve the immune system. Adding fresh garlic or garlic powder to food can make it taste better and help the body heal after surgery.

using healing herbs and spices in your post-surgery diet can help in many ways, such as lowering inflammation, improving digestion, and making food taste better. People who are having rectal surgery can speed up their recovery and improve their health in the long run by adding anti-inflammatory foods, digestive-helping herbs, and flavorful spice blends to their meals.

Additionally, talking to a doctor or nutritionist can give you specific advice on how to effectively include these foods in your diet.

CHAPTER 10
MEAL PLANS AND EXAMPLE MENU

When it comes to eating for recovering from rectal surgery, making a full meal plan that fits each person's needs is very important for speeding up the healing process, building strength, and avoiding problems. A well-thought-out meal plan not only makes sure that you get enough food but also speeds up the healing process. Let's talk about how to make meal plans and sample menus that are perfect for people who have recently had abdominal surgery.

Menus for each week

Making a weekly meal plan gives you order and consistency, which are both important for a smooth recovery process. To help tissues heal and the immune system work better, a well-balanced meal plan should include a range of nutrients, such as proteins, carbs, healthy fats, vitamins, and minerals. It's important to eat a lot of nutrient-dense foods and not too many processed or toxic ones. Planning meals ahead of time not only makes grocery shopping easier but also makes it easier to stick to dietary rules, which is good for recovery.

When planning your weekly meals, you might want to include foods from a lot of different food groups to make sure you get all the nutrients you need. Eat a variety of foods to get the right amount of lean proteins, complex carbohydrates, and healthy fats. Lean proteins include chicken, fish, tofu, and legumes. Complex carbohydrates include whole grains, fruits, and veggies. Also, make sure you eat a lot of fiber to keep your bowel movements regular and avoid constipation, which is a typical problem after rectal surgery. Adding probiotic-rich foods like yogurt, kefir, and fermented veggies to your diet can also help your gut stay healthy and your digestion.

Daily meal plans should be based on the principles of proper nutrition and take into account each person's tastes and dietary needs. For breakfast, you could have muesli with fresh berries and almonds on top, whole-grain toast with avocado and poached eggs, or a drink made with spinach, banana, Greek yogurt, and flaxseeds.

For lunch, you could have a salad with mixed greens, grilled chicken or salmon, quinoa, and different coloured veggies that have been drizzled with olive oil and balsamic vinegar. You could also eat hearty soups or sandwiches made with whole-grain bread, lean meats, and lots of vegetables.

You can get lean protein for dinner by baking fish or tofu and serving it with brown rice, roasted vegetables, and lentil stew with sweet potatoes and kale. You can also get stir-fried veggies with lean beef or prawns over whole-wheat noodles.

Healthy snacks are good for you and make you feel full, like a handful of nuts and seeds, Greek yogurt with fruit, or hummus and veggie sticks.

Also, staying hydrated is important for healing, so make sure you drink enough water throughout the day and avoid sugary drinks and too much caffeine.

Making changes to dietary restrictions

When making meal plans for people who have had abdominal surgery, it's important to take into account any food allergies or limits they may have. Some people may need to stay away from certain foods that could make stomach problems worse or cause the medicine to not work right. People who are sensitive to lactose, for example, can choose dairy products that don't contain lactose.

People who are sensitive to gluten, on the other hand, should choose grains that don't contain gluten, such as rice, quinoa, and buckwheat.

Also, people who are having rectal surgery may need to make brief changes to their diets depending on their medical condition or surgery.

For example, people who have a colostomy or an ileostomy may need to change what they eat to control the flow of their ostomy and avoid problems like blockages or becoming dehydrated.

When this happens, it's important to work closely with a qualified dietitian or healthcare provider to make sure you get enough nutrition and recover as quickly as possible.

Finally, making meal plans and example menus that are specific to the needs of people who have had abdominal surgery is a very important part of helping them recover and stay healthy in the long term.

Healthcare professionals can give people the tools they need to make healthy decisions that help them heal and improve their quality of life by focusing on nutrient-rich foods, offering a variety of meal options, and working with dietary restrictions. Good nutrition after surgery not only speeds up the healing process but also sets the stage for long-term health and energy.

CHAPTER 11
HELPING YOU ON YOUR WAY TO RECOVERY

Recovery from rectal surgery is a very important time that needs careful attention to many things, such as diet. During the time after surgery, the body needs the best diet to heal tissues, boost the immune system, and improve health in general. This complete guide to the best diet after surgery for people who have just been identified goes into detail about the most important parts of using food to help with recovery. It includes healing recipes, meal plans, and expert advice for long-term health.

Care for Yourself While You're Healing

Taking care of yourself is very important during the healing process after rectal surgery. It means consciously taking care of your physical, emotional, and mental needs to help you heal and improve your general health.

Following a healthy, well-balanced diet designed to help the body heal is an important part of taking care of yourself while you're recovering.

 To do this, you need to eat foods that are high in nutrients, like vitamins, minerals, protein, and fiber, which are all important for healing tissues and keeping your immune system healthy. Also, staying refreshed is important to avoid becoming dehydrated, keep organs working well, and make it easier for the body to get rid of toxins.

Making sure you get enough rest and sleep is another important part of self-care while you're recovering. The body needs enough rest to heal from the stress of surgery and recover from its effects. Setting a regular sleep routine and making your bedroom more comfortable can help you get better sleep, which is important for your overall recovery. Using relaxation methods like deep breathing, meditation, or gentle stretching can also help reduce stress and promote relaxation, which can speed up the healing process.

During the recovery time, it's also good to do light physical activity as tolerated. It's important to stay away from activities that are too hard on tissues that are still healing, but light movements like short walks or light stretching exercises can help circulation, lower the risk of complications like blood clots, and improve general health. But it's very important to do what the doctors tell you and slowly increase your exercise level based on how well you're recovering.

Putting together a support system

Having a strong network of support is very helpful when you are recovering from rectal surgery.

A person's support system could include family, friends, healthcare experts, and support groups. These people offer emotional support, practical help, and motivation as the person recovers.

Telling your loved ones about your needs, worries, and progress in an honest way can help you feel connected and less alone or anxious.

In addition to personal support networks, it can be helpful to use expert support services while you are recovering. This could mean working with a registered dietitian to make a personalised nutrition plan, talking to a physical therapist about safe rehabilitation exercises, or going to counseling or psychotherapy to deal with emotional or mental problems that come up during surgery and recovery.

How to Stay Positive and Motivated

Having a positive attitude and staying focused is very important during recovery from rectal surgery. It's normal to have changes in mood and feelings while you're healing, but keeping a positive attitude can help you stay strong and make progress toward your recovery goals. Doing things that make you happy and fulfilled, like hobbies, spending time with loved ones, or practicing gratitude, can lift your mood and improve your mental health.

Making goals that are attainable and enjoying small wins along the way can also help you stay motivated and on track while you're recovering. Taking on bigger jobs one step at a time and keeping track of your progress can help you feel accomplished and in control. A feeling of control and independence can also be gained by staying informed about the recovery process, asking questions, and taking an active role in making decisions about treatment and self-care.

Adding mindfulness techniques like mindful eating or mindfulness meditation to your daily life can help you feel better overall, lower your stress, and concentrate better. People can become more resilient to dealing with problems and setbacks along the way to healing by staying in the present moment and becoming more aware of their thoughts, feelings, and body sensations.

Taking a whole-person approach to recovery from rectal surgery, which includes taking care of yourself, making friends, and keeping an upbeat attitude, is important. People can speed up their recovery and set themselves up for long-term health by putting nutrition, rest, physical exercise, and emotional health at the top of their list of priorities. People can get through the tough parts of recovery with strength and determination if they know themselves, keep going, and get help from family, friends, and medical experts.

CONCLUSION

Getting the right diet is very important for healing after rectal surgery. This complete guide has taught me a lot about how important diet is during this very important time.

People can help their recovery process by learning about the details of rectal surgery, making sure their kitchen is well-stocked, and eating foods that are high in nutrients.

The chapters talked about different kinds of meals that could help people at different points of their recovery. These included soups and soft dishes that are good for you, as well as meals that are high in protein and fiber.

 It was important to stay hydrated, keep your electrolytes in balance, and use healing herbs and spices to improve your general health.

Also, giving people meal plans, sample recipes, and advice on how to work around dietary restrictions makes sure that they can easily and confidently follow their post-surgery diet.

It was also emphasized how important it is to take care of yourself, build a support system, and keep an upbeat attitude during recovery.

People who are getting rectal surgery can improve their diet after surgery, speed up the healing process, and set themselves up for long-term health and vitality by following the experts' advice and using the resources given.

This book is a complete resource for people who want to improve their health after rectal surgery. It includes healing recipes, meal plans, and expert advice for a smooth recovery.